Anatomy Digestive & Endocrine System Label Practice

By K.R. Lefkowitz

ISBN: 10:1532998848
ISBN-13: 978-1532998843

DIGESTIVE & ENDOCRINE SYSTEM

How To Use....

This book is mean't to be used for you to label and practice the components of the Digestive & Endocrine system. In going through your anatomy class and later in medical field you will need to know how to label the components, pictures of each system and know it inside and out. The best way is for you to label all the components that you know yourself and research the areas that you don't. Can you label all parts of the muscles, both deep and superficial, etc...? Can you recognize a picture and know immediately what it is? You can find the corresponding picture in the table of contents. Nothing is labeled on purpose. This is for you to label. For you to know. And what you don't know for you to research in your texts and find the answers. Through this way of learning and researching the parts you don't know, allows you to actually learn it and have it stored in long term memory. This active way of learning will in the long term be beneficial beyond belief in your future career or knowledge. Mark the pages, make notes, and use this practice book and pictures to help you understand the parts of the anatomy.

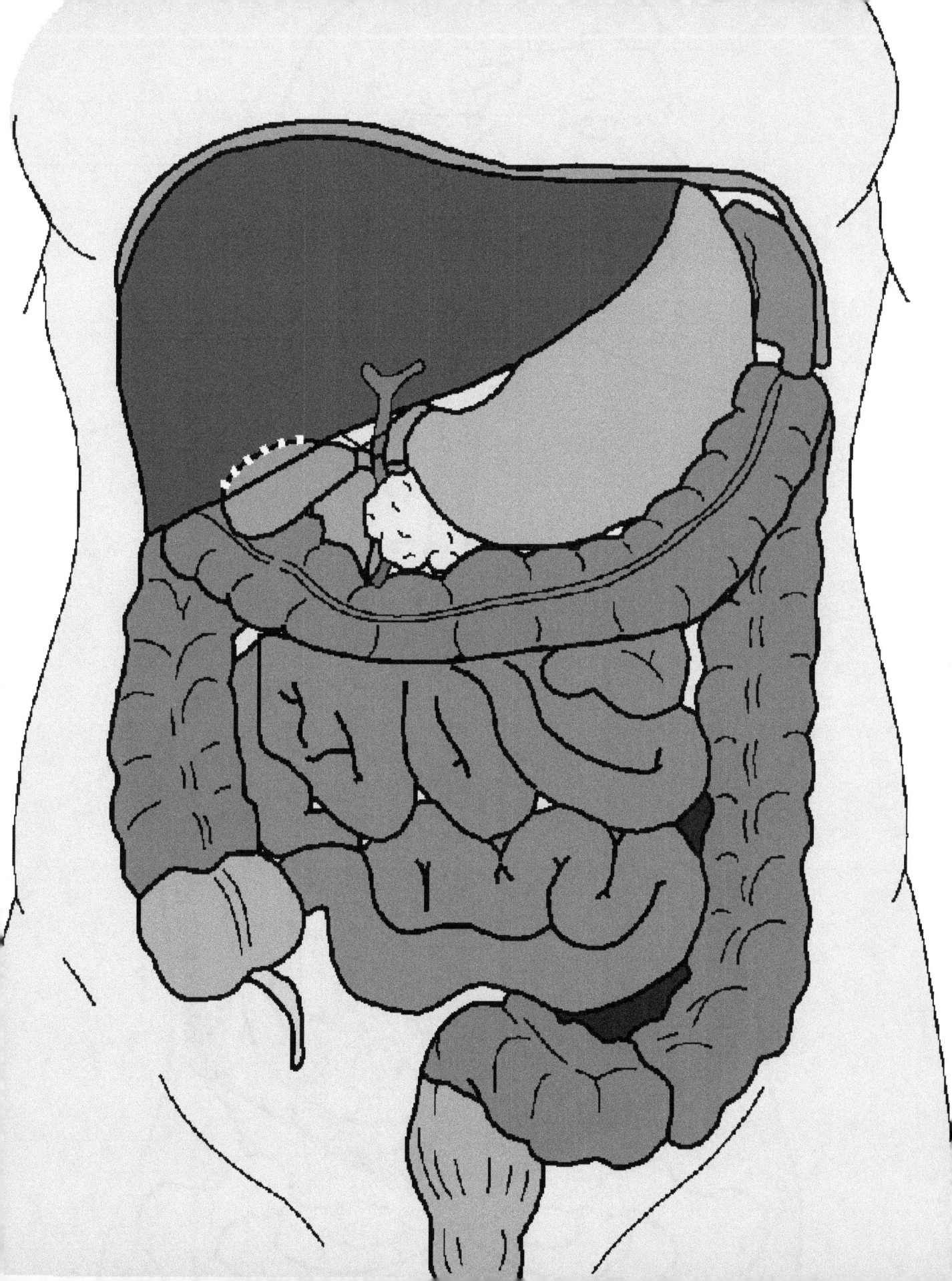

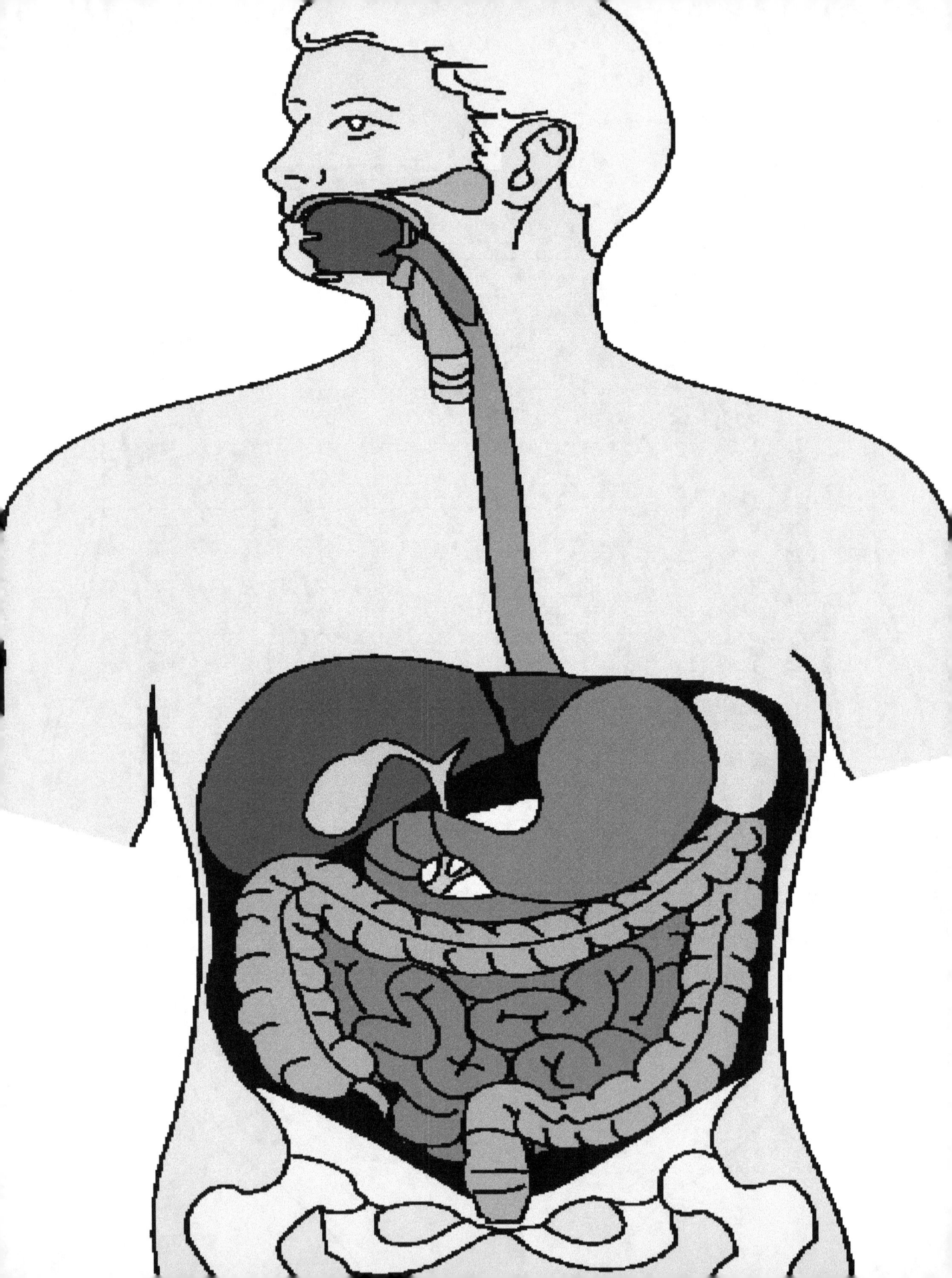

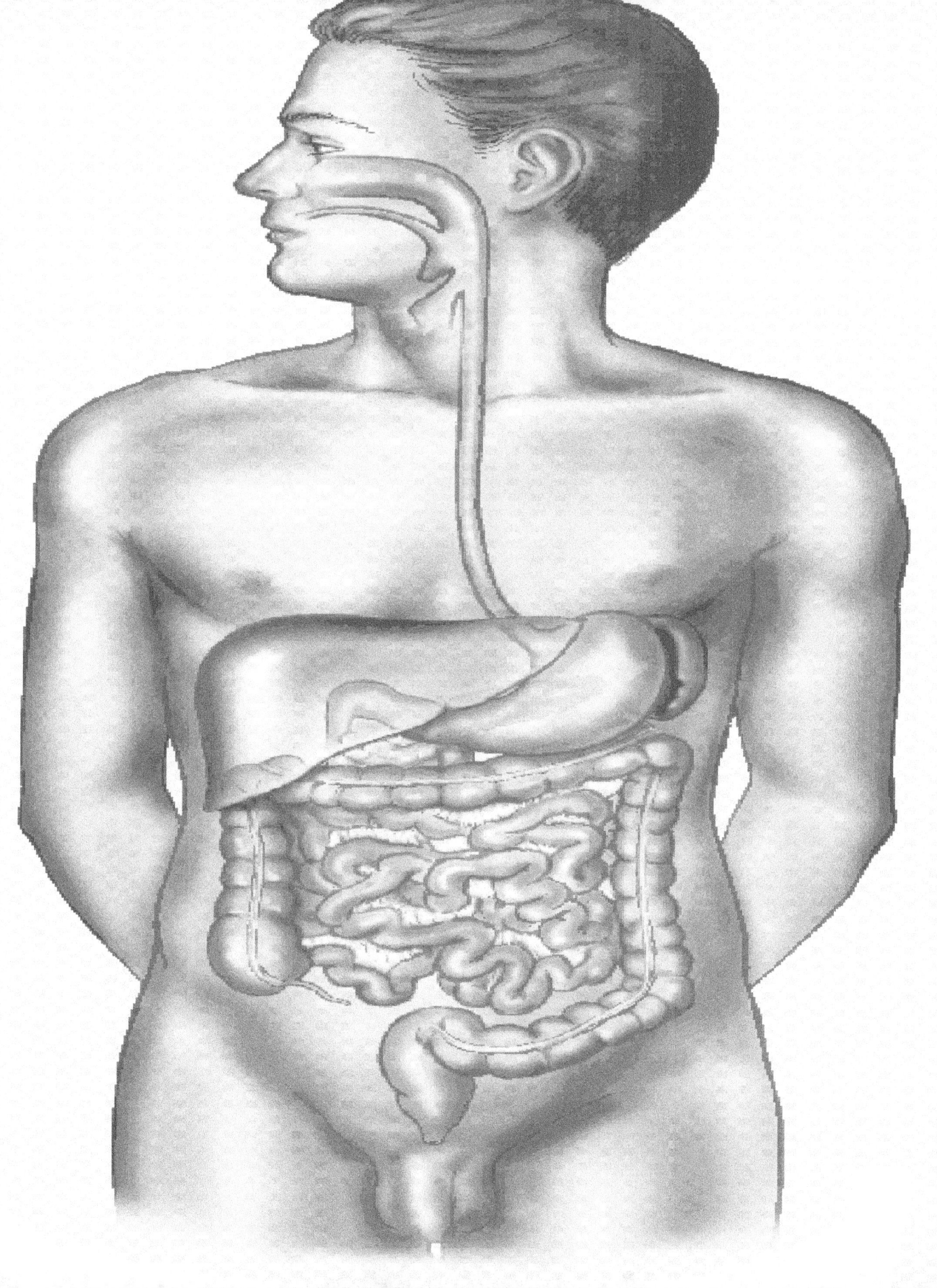

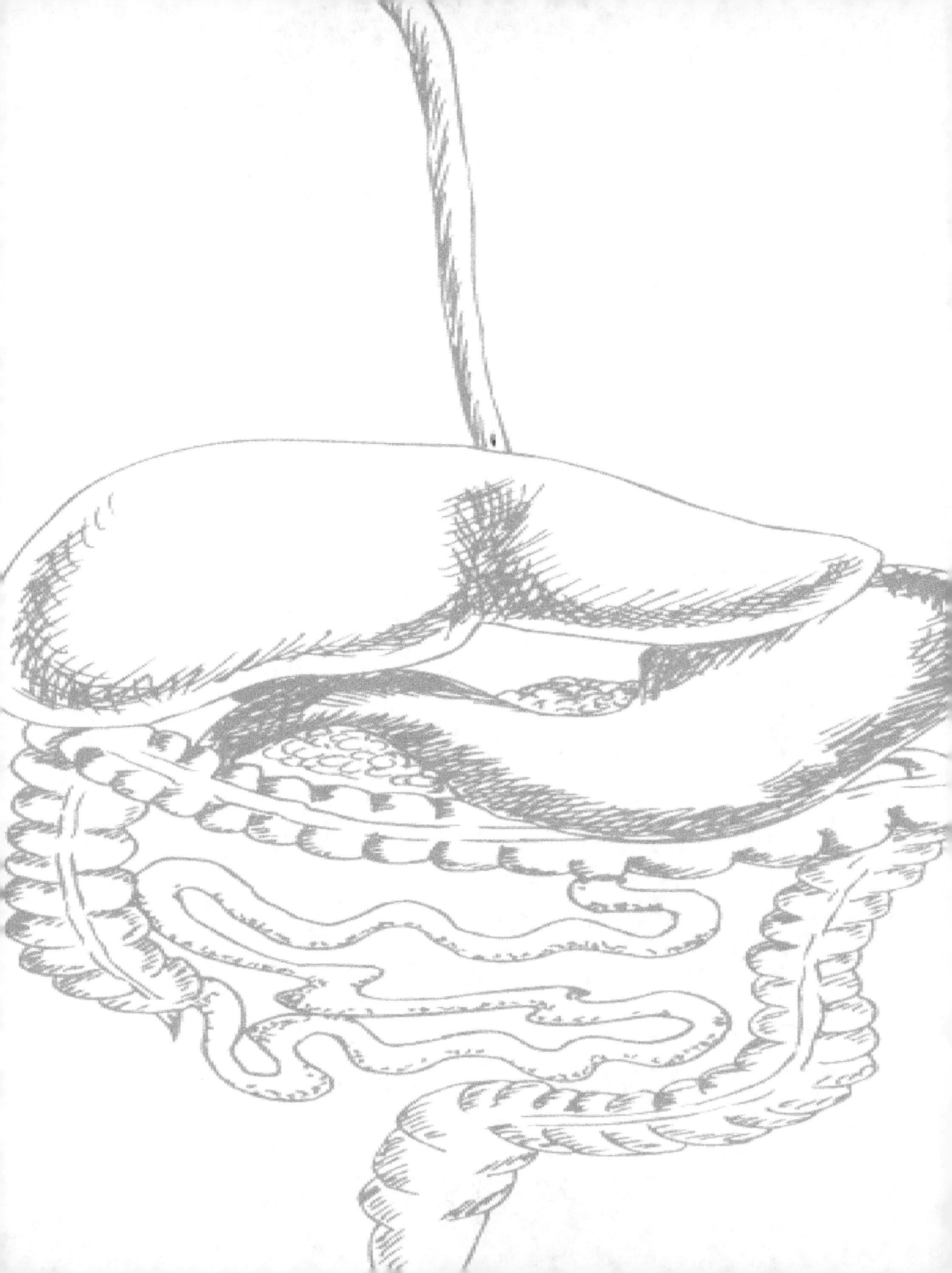

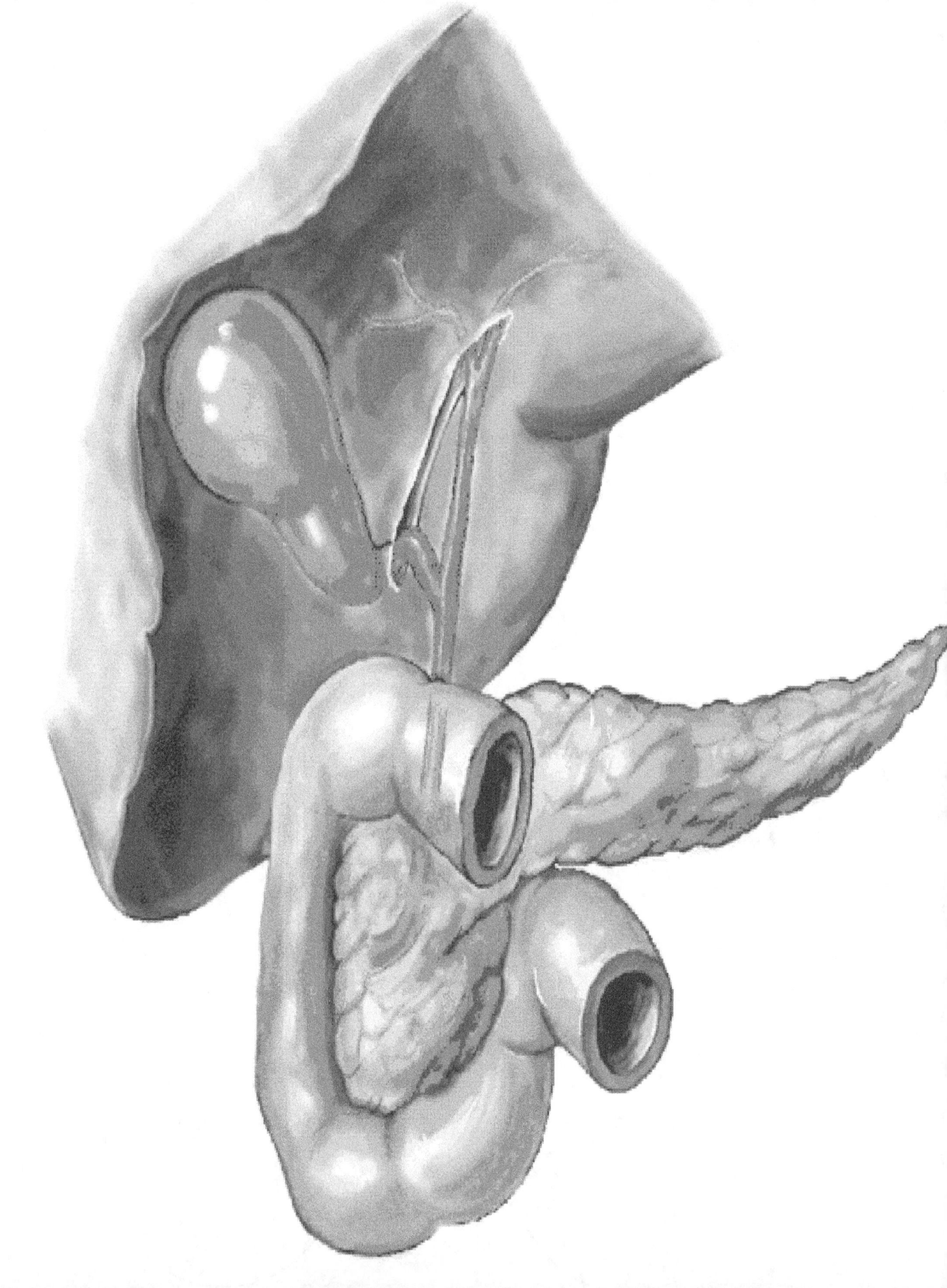

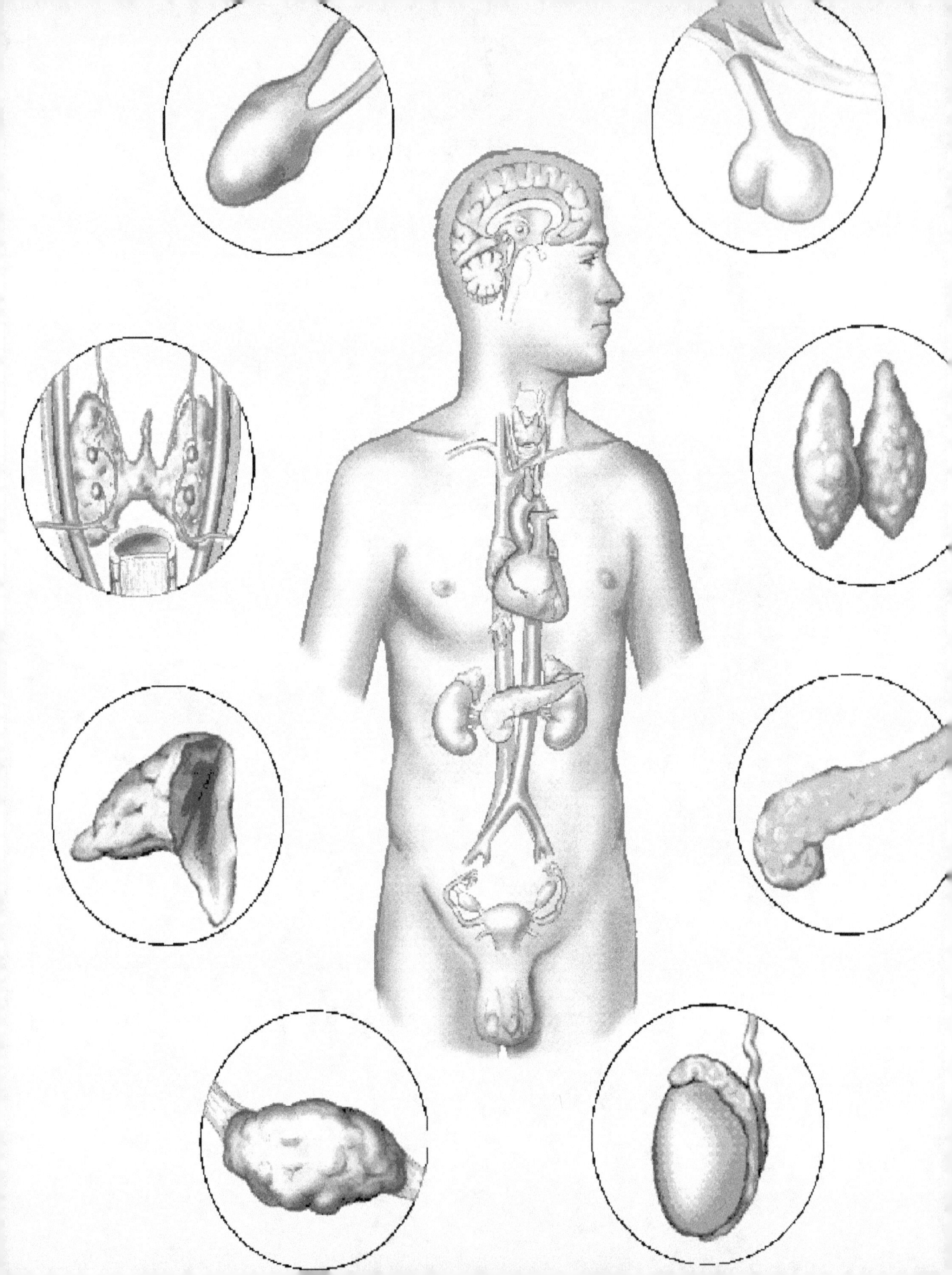

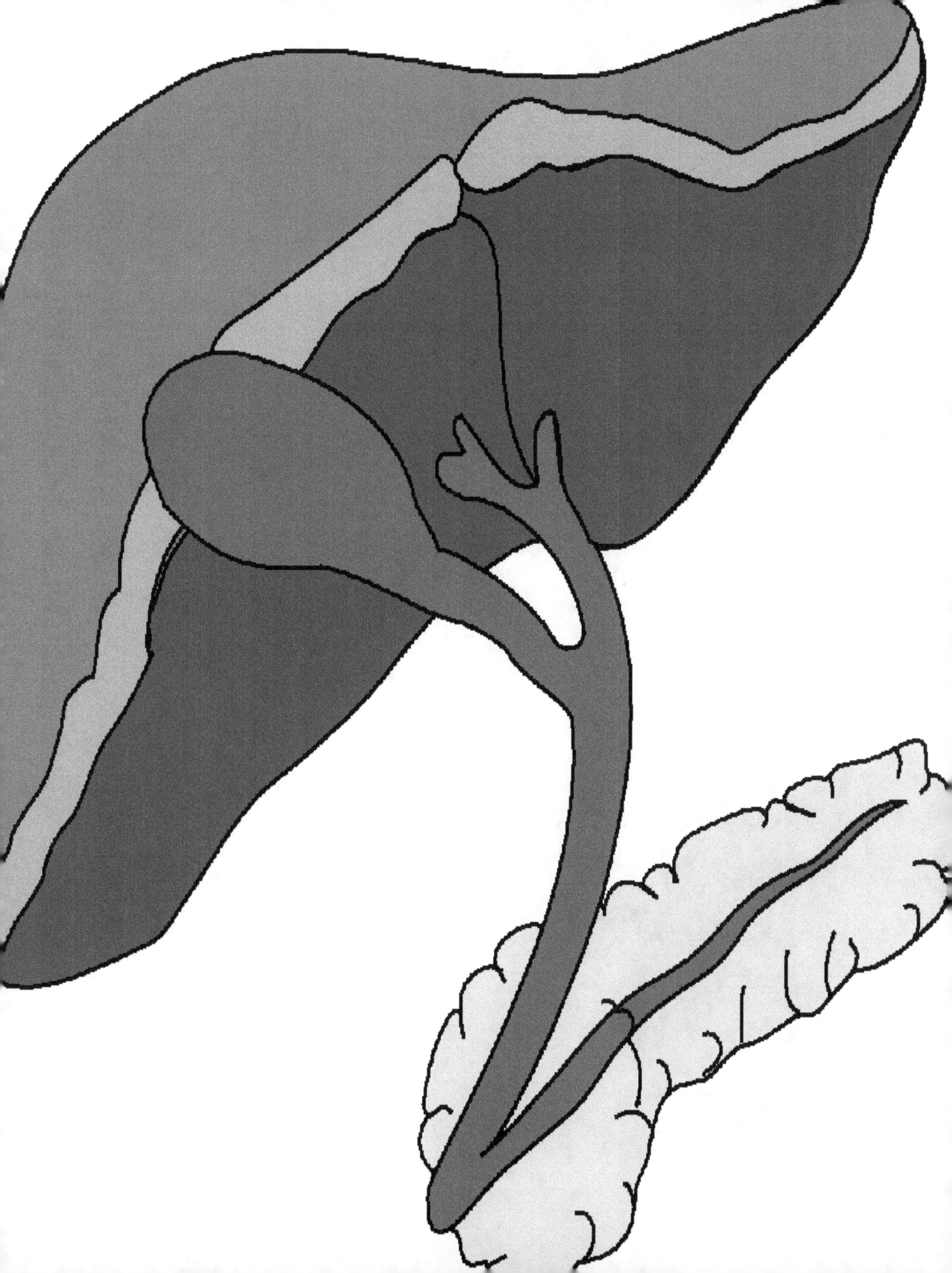

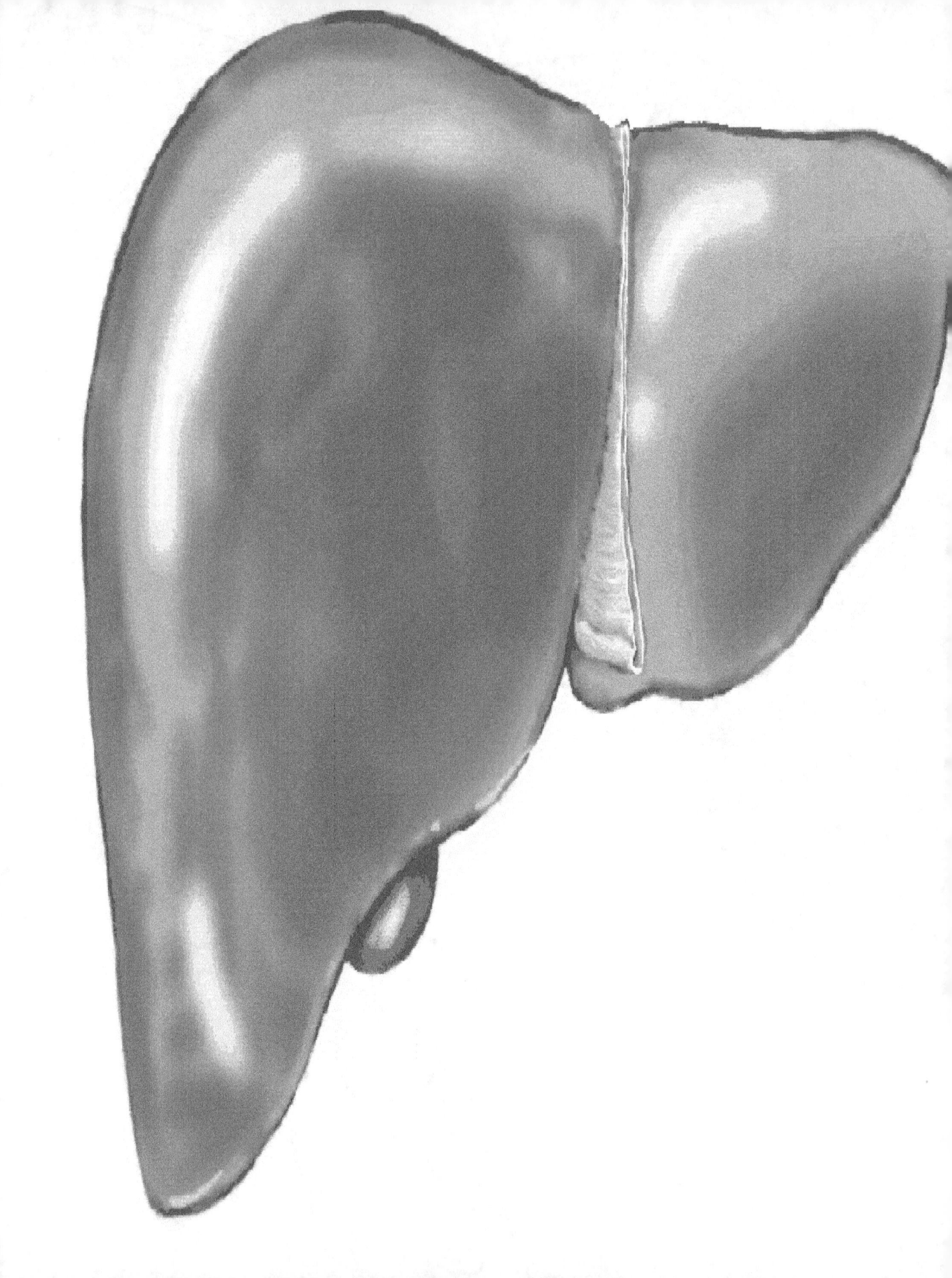

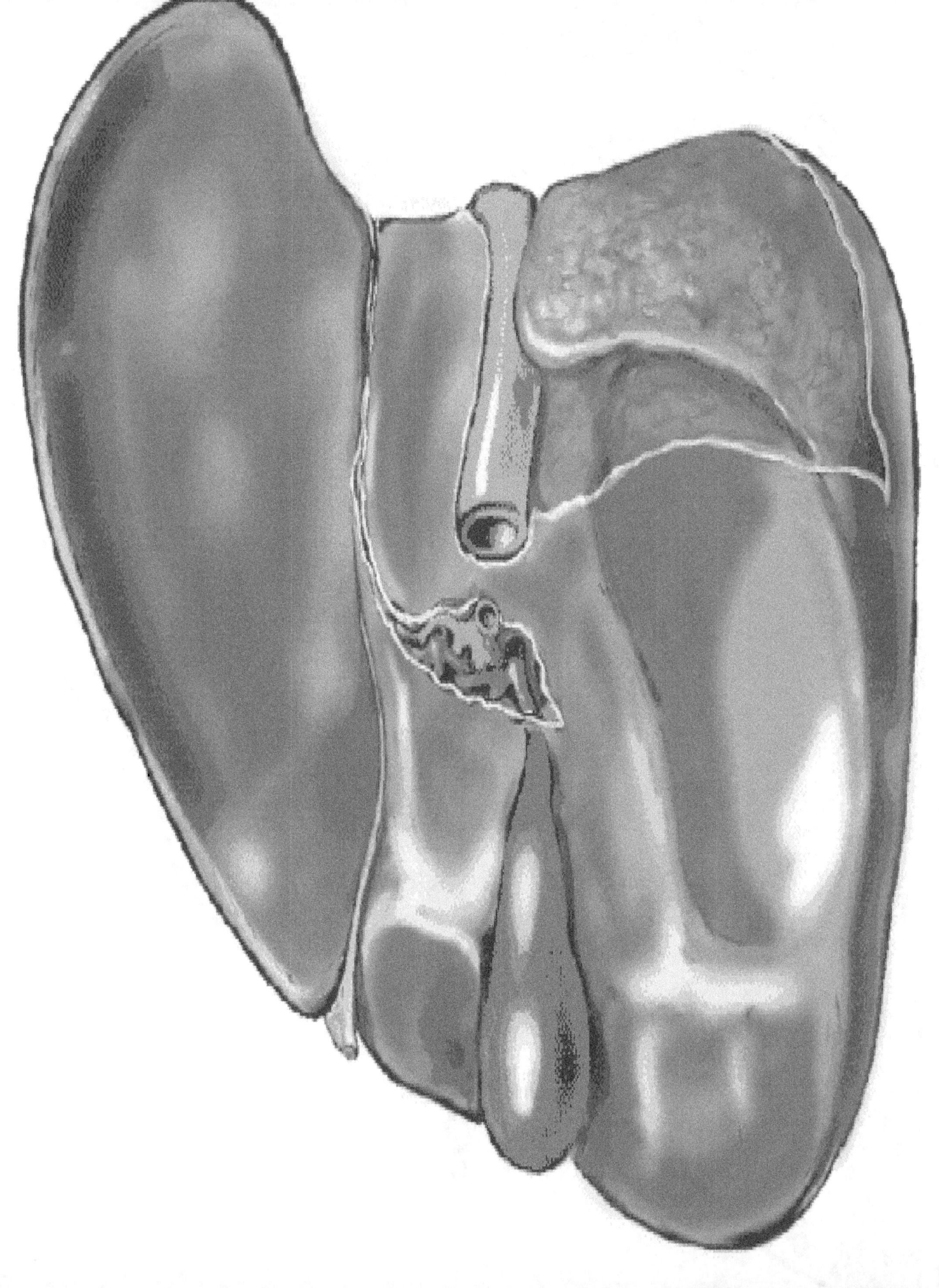

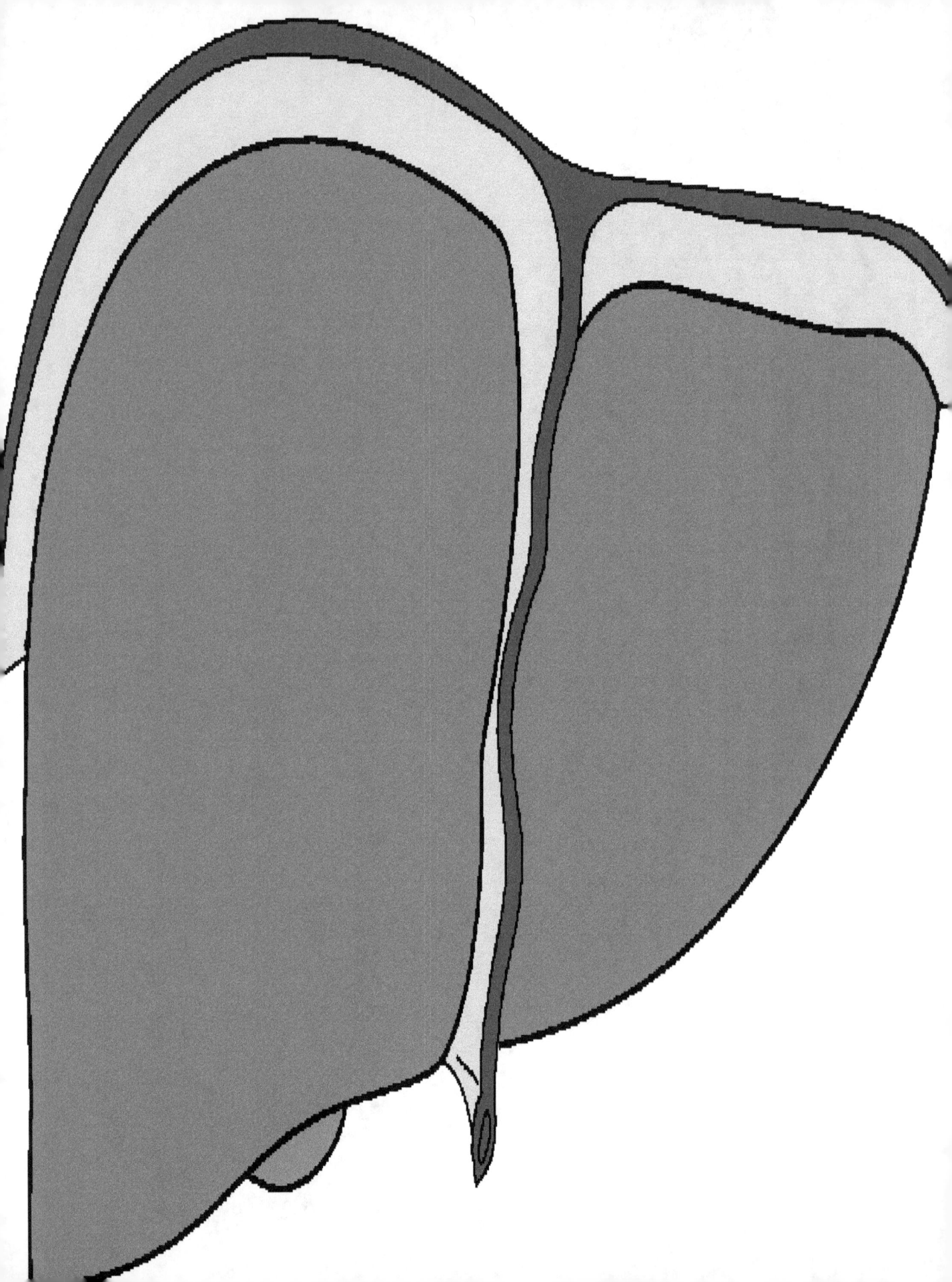

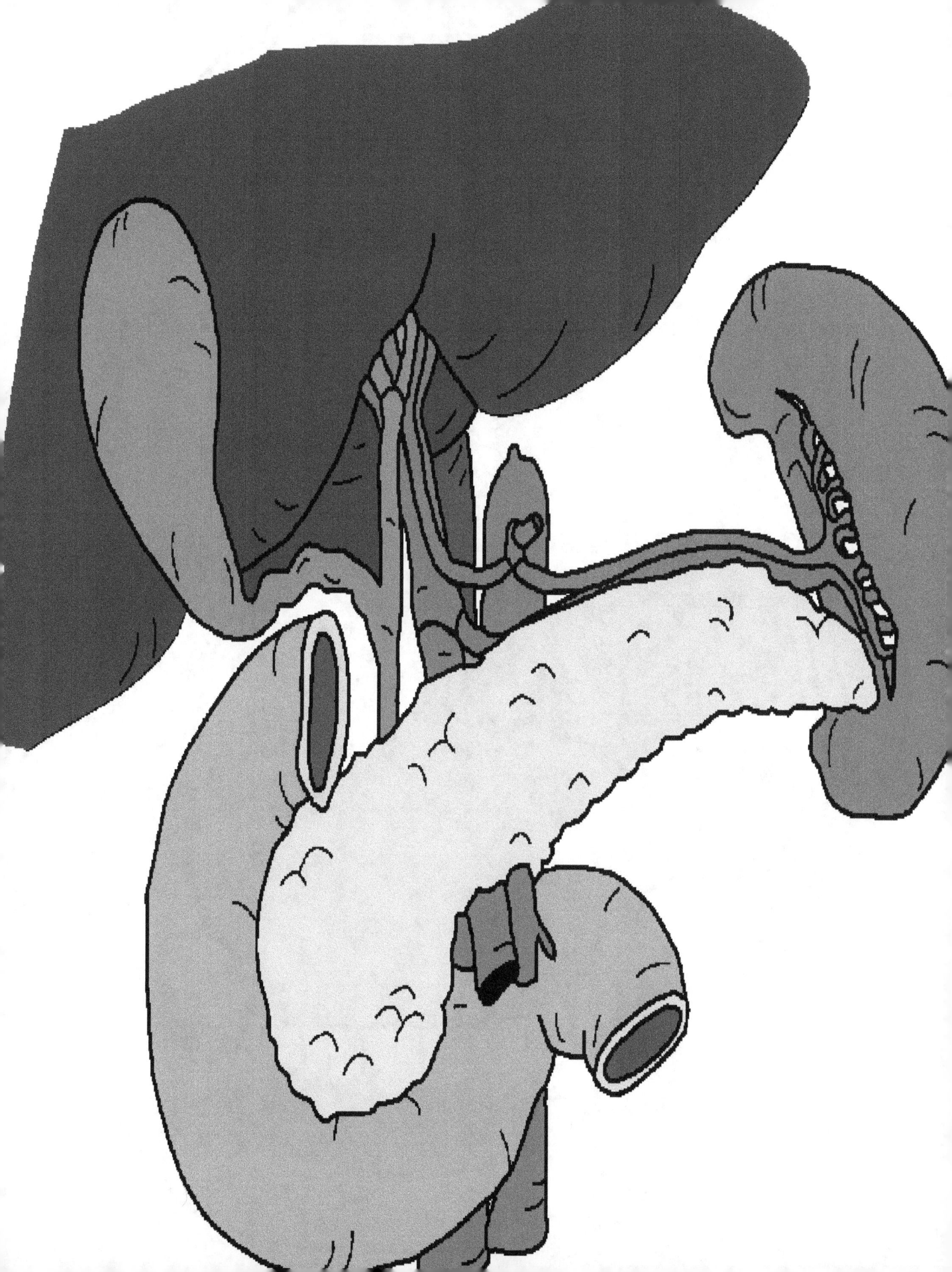

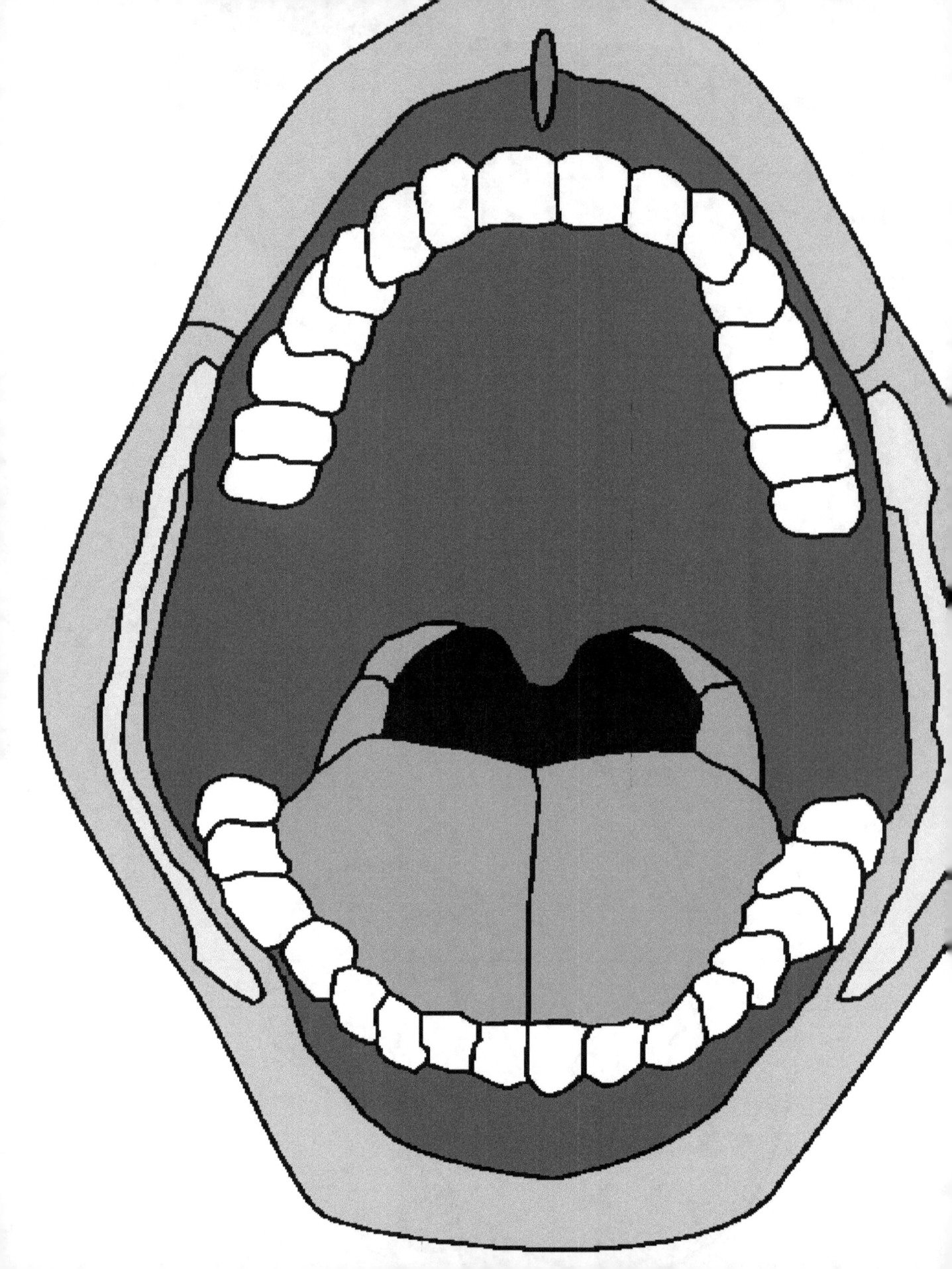

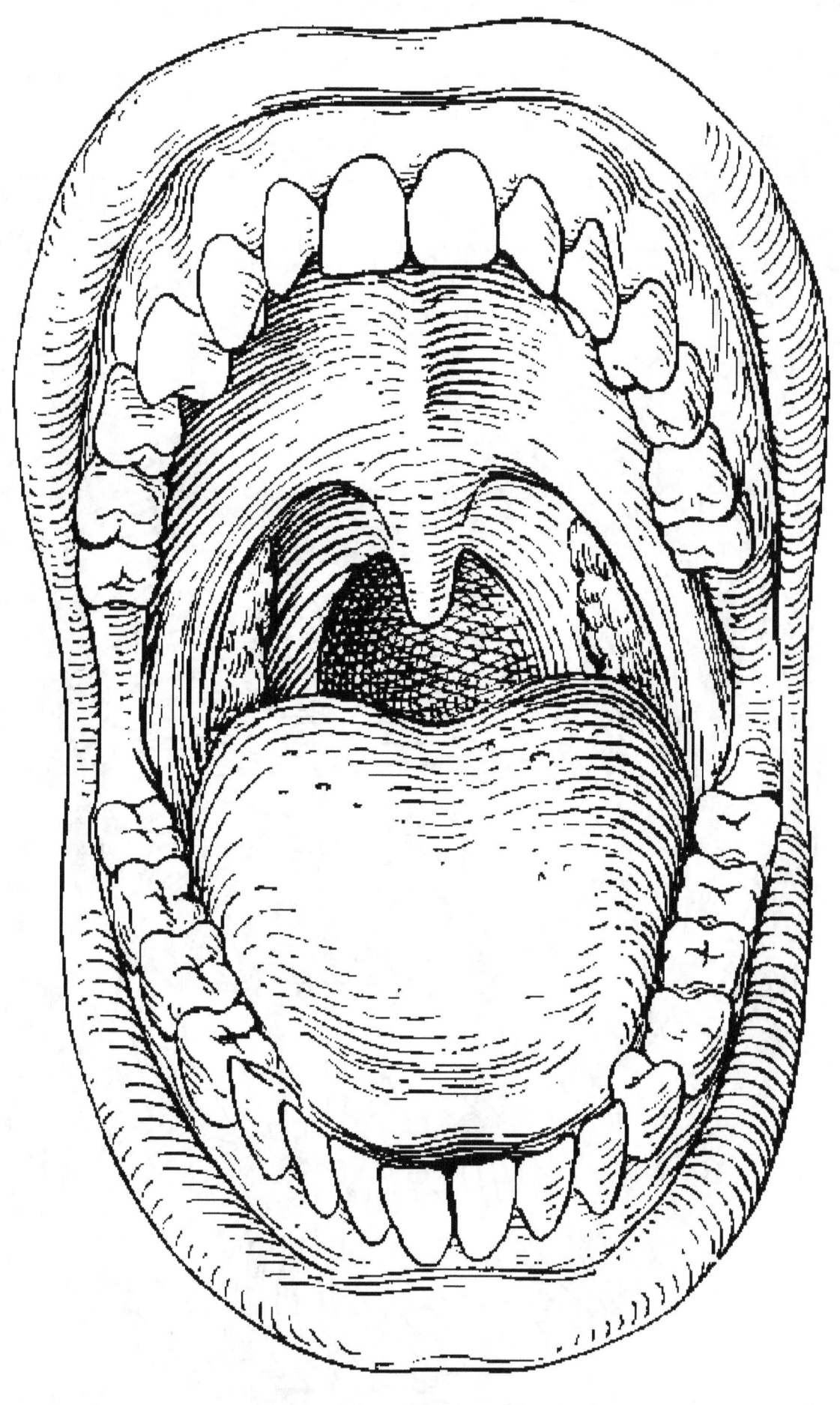

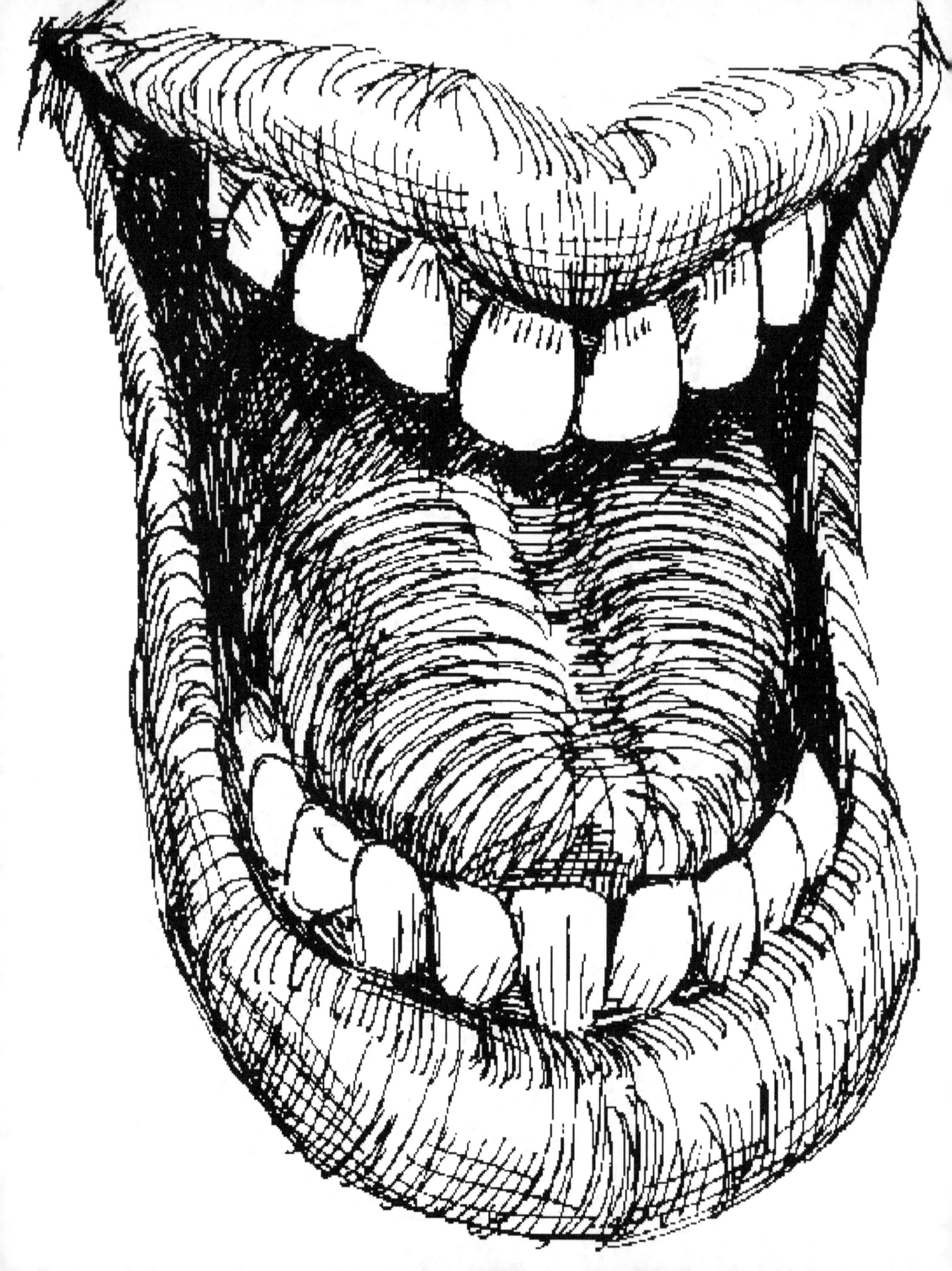

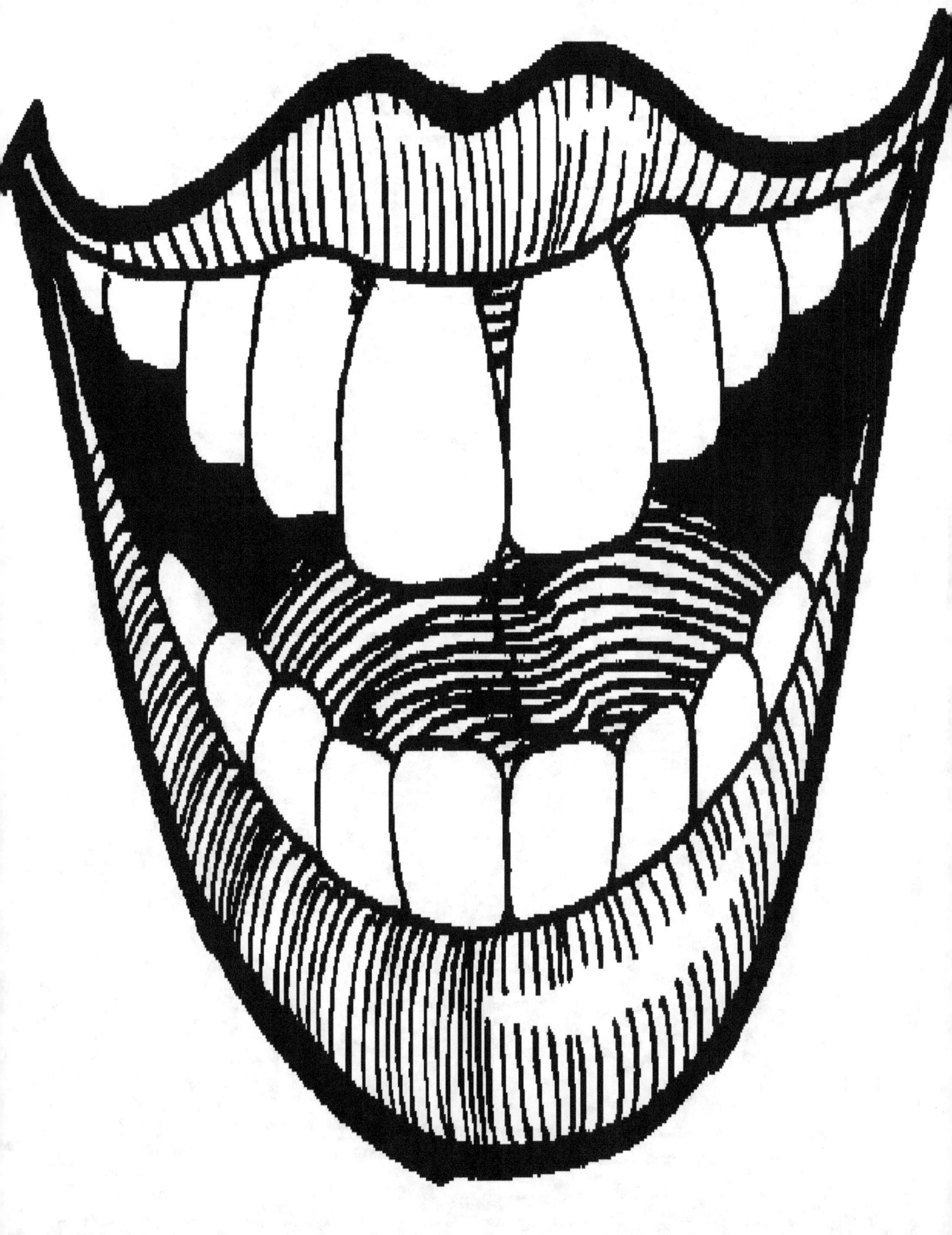

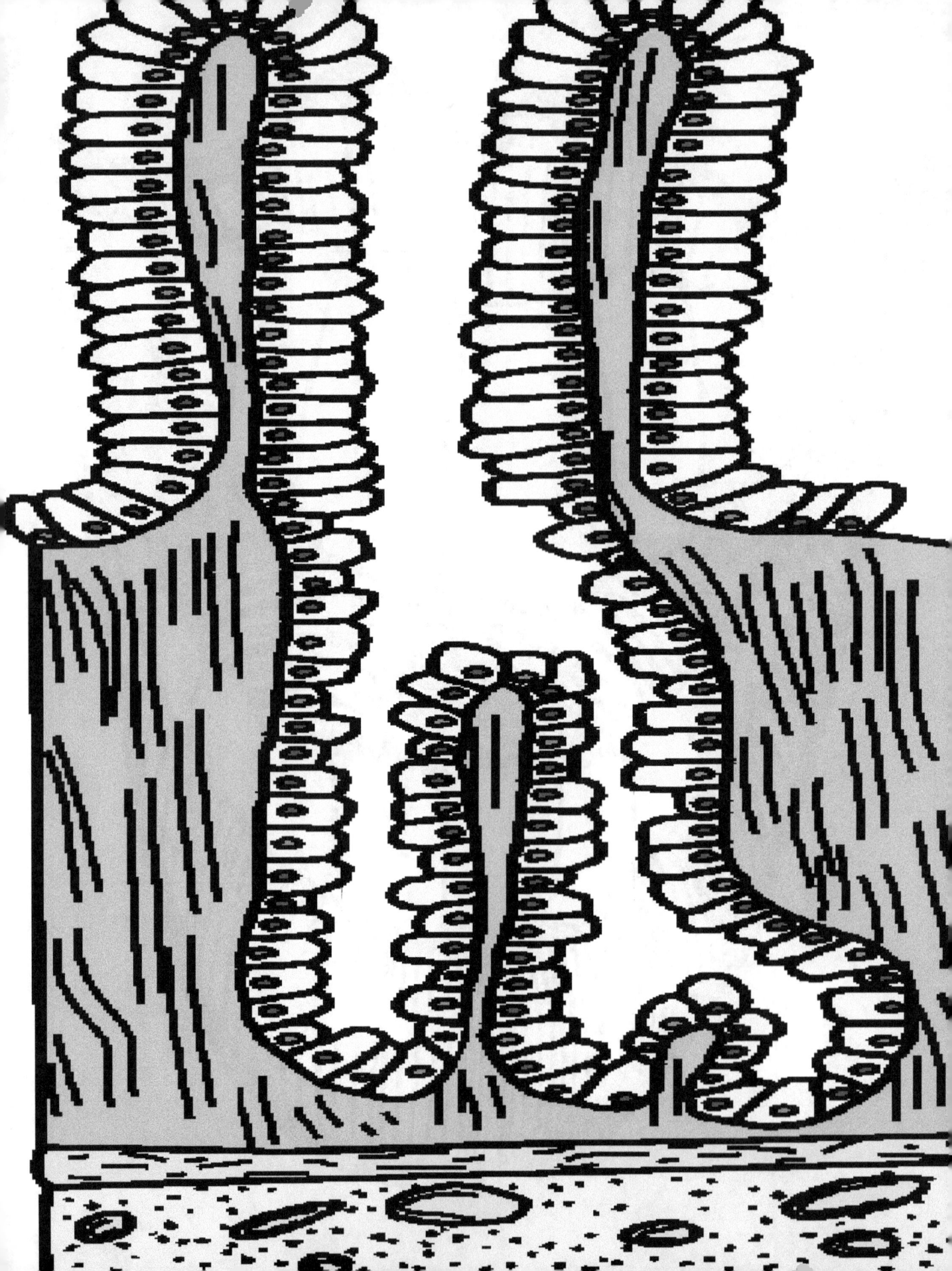

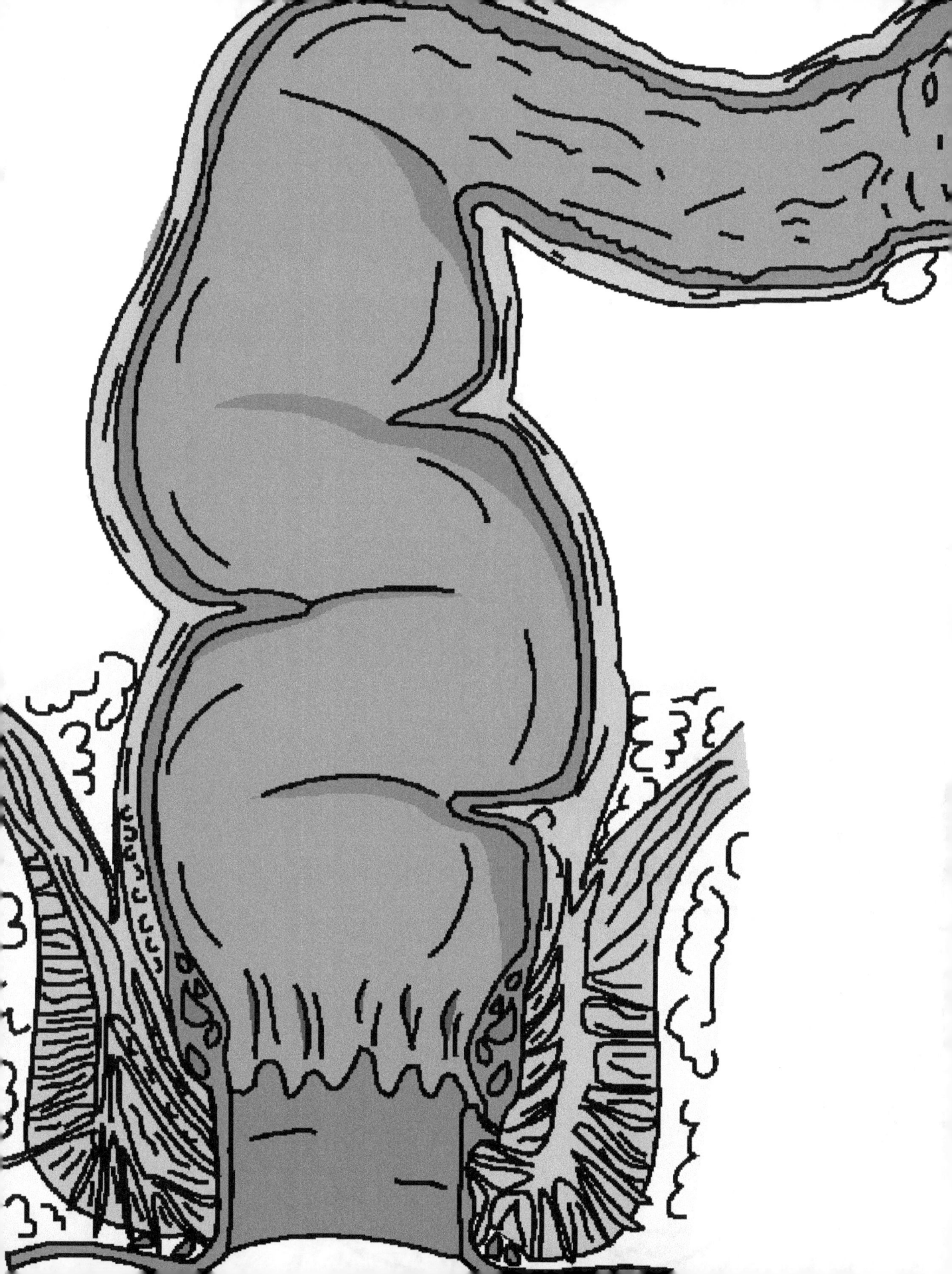

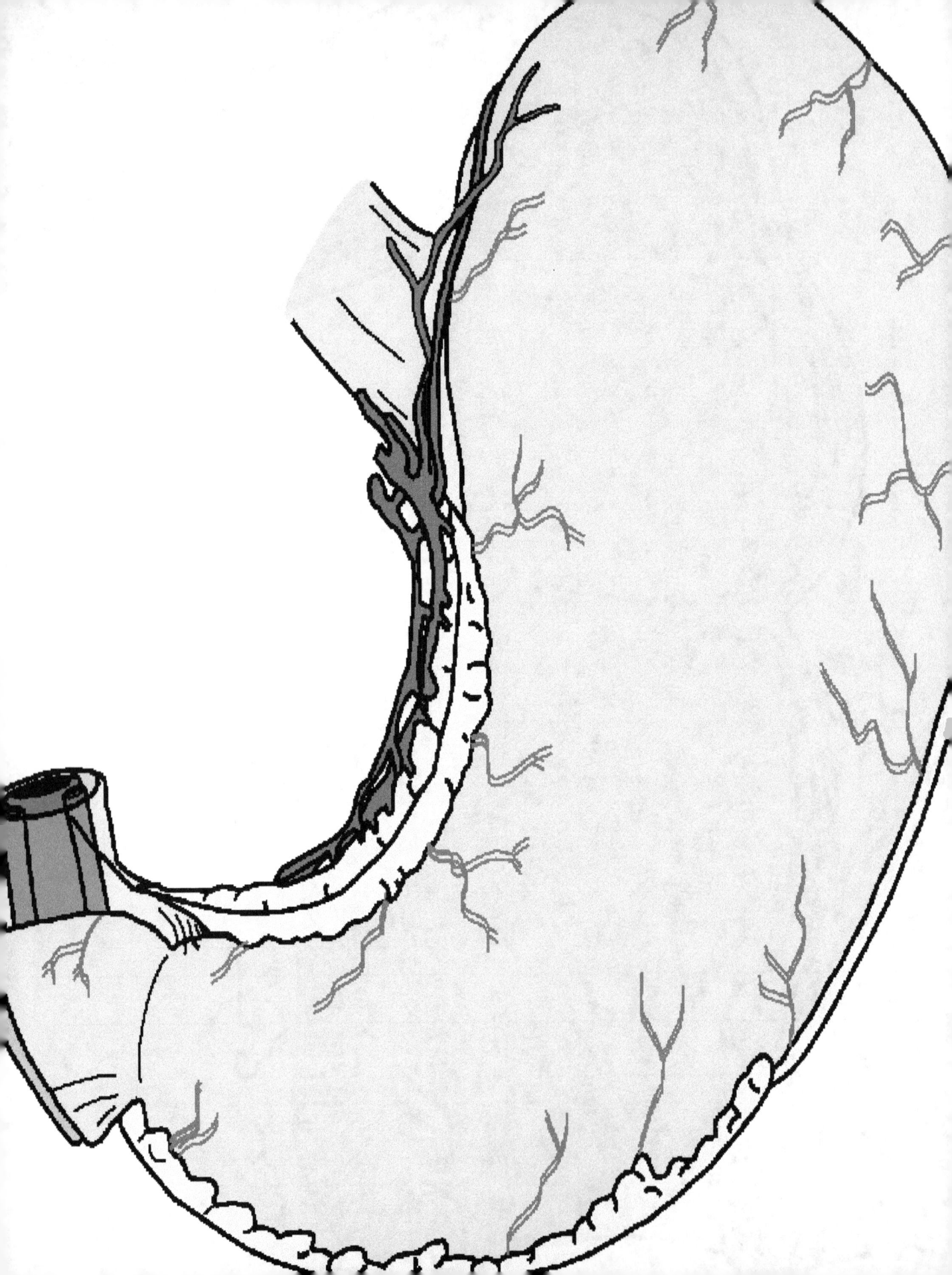

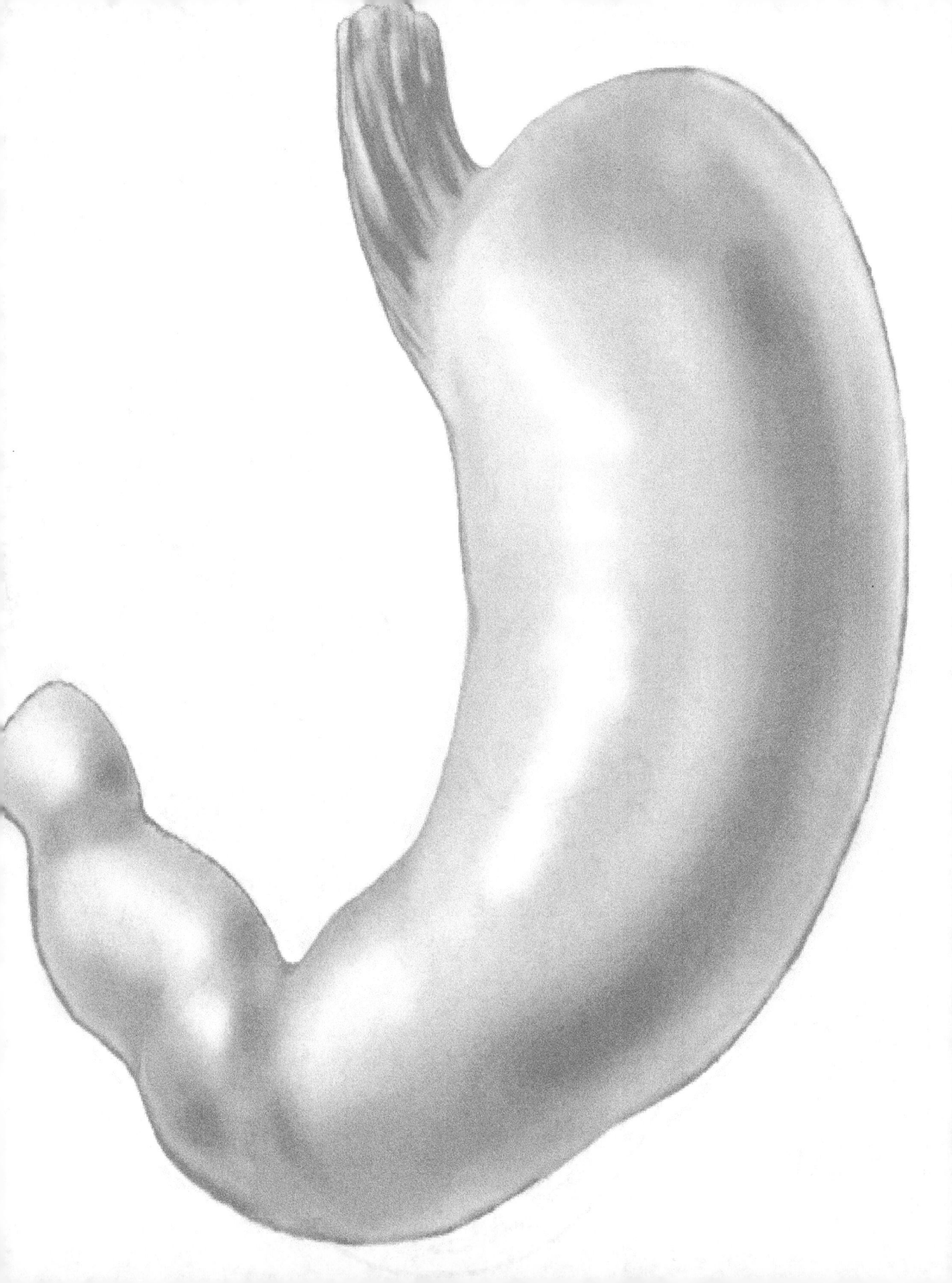

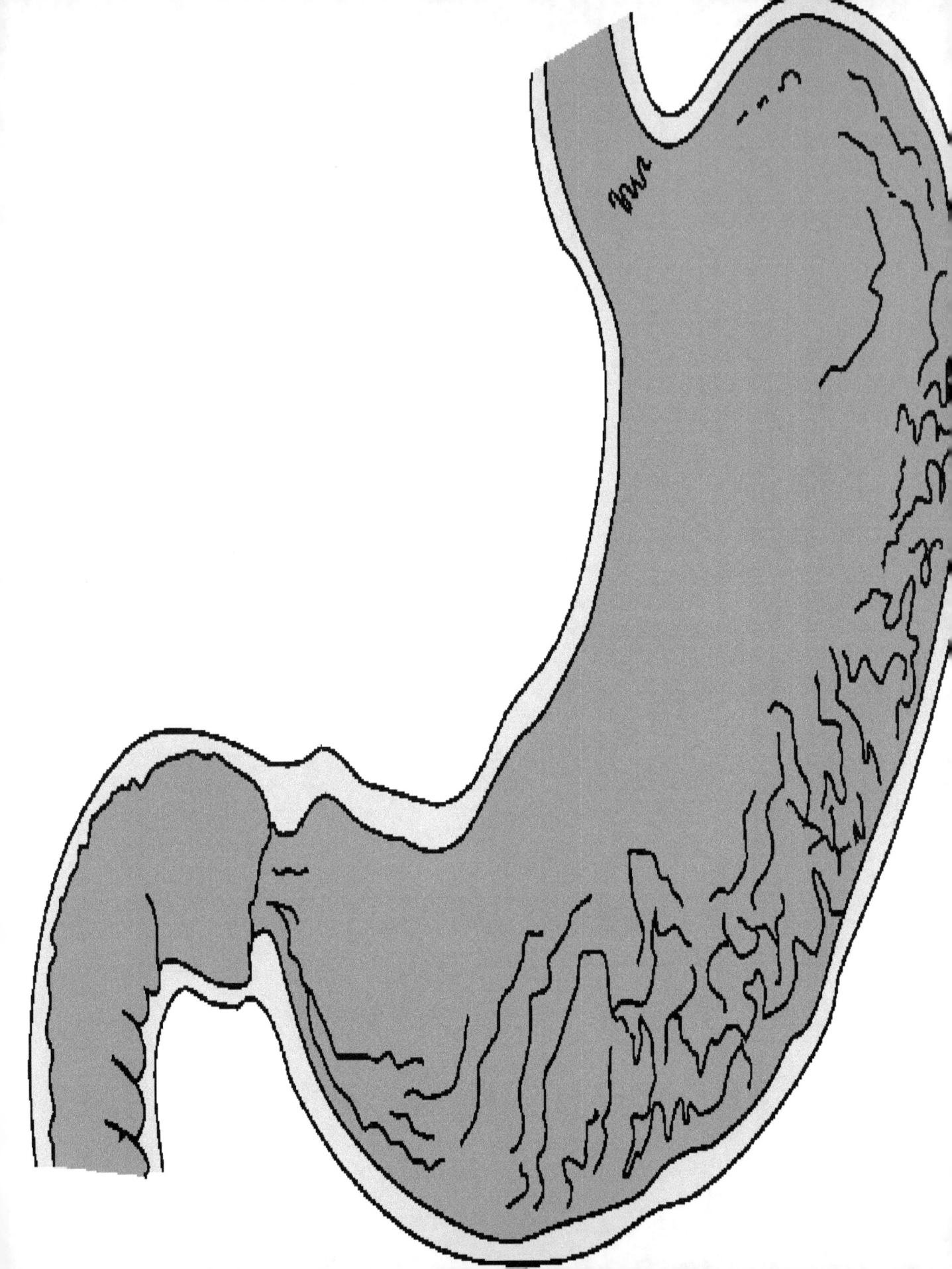

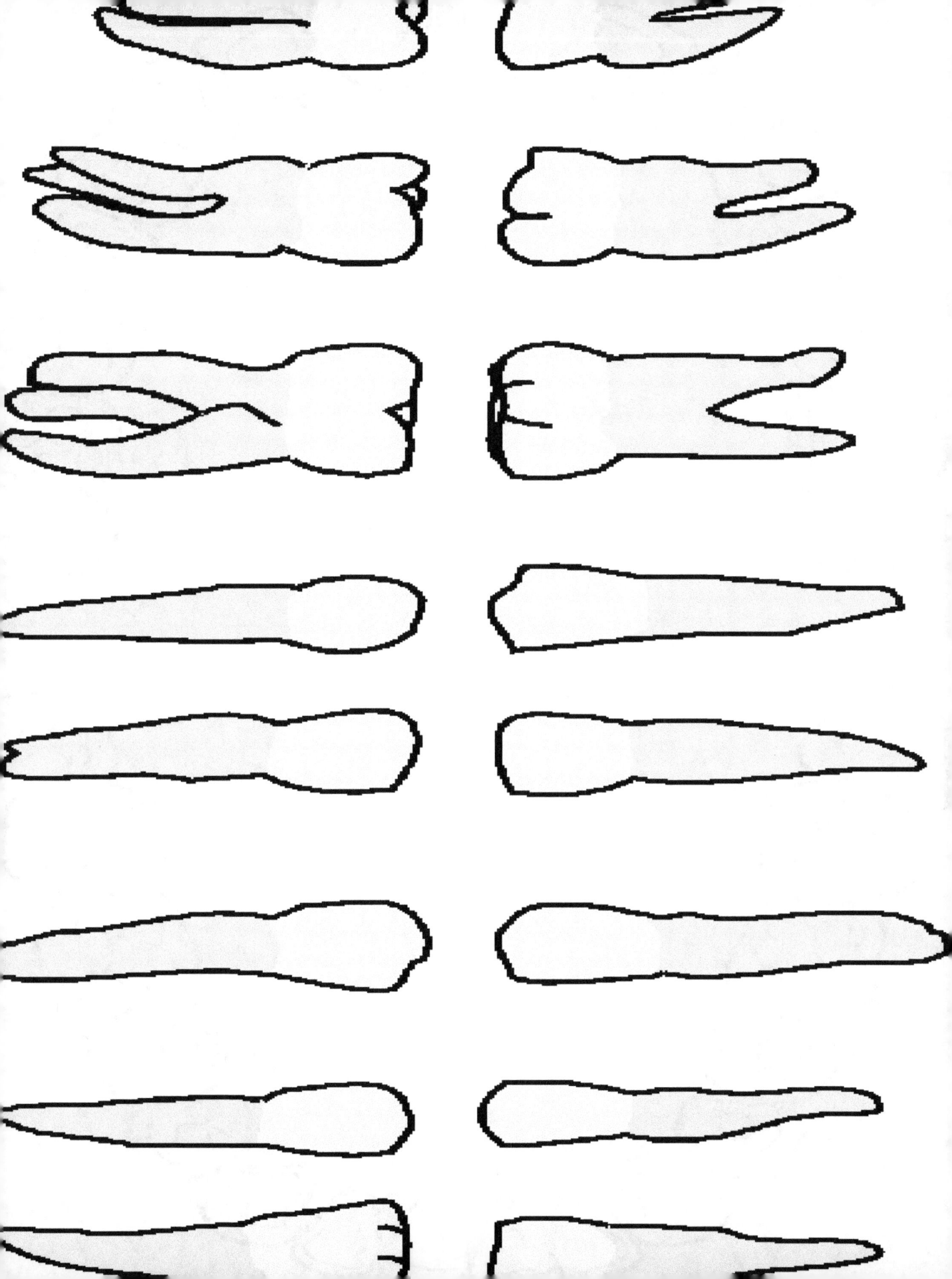

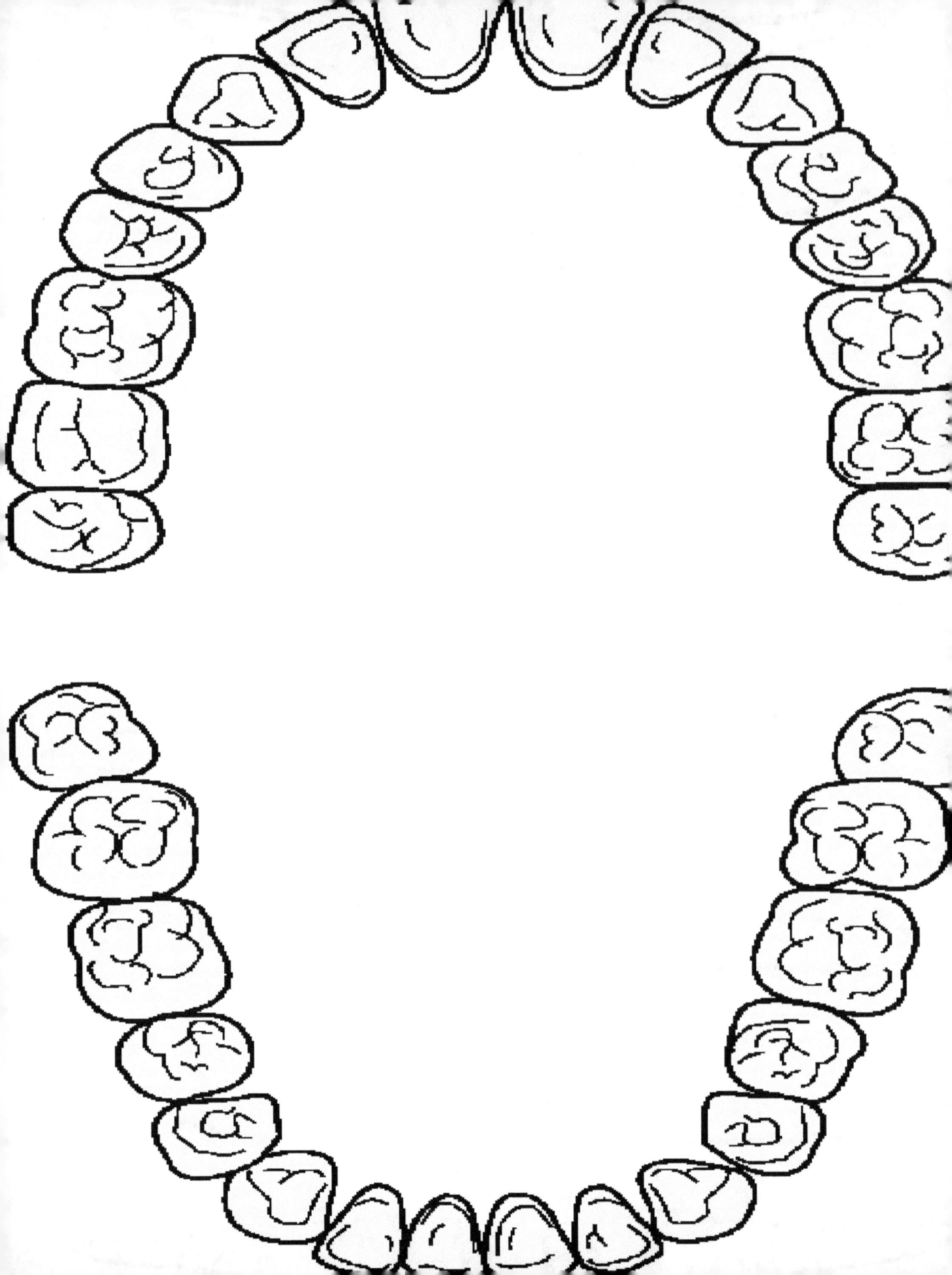

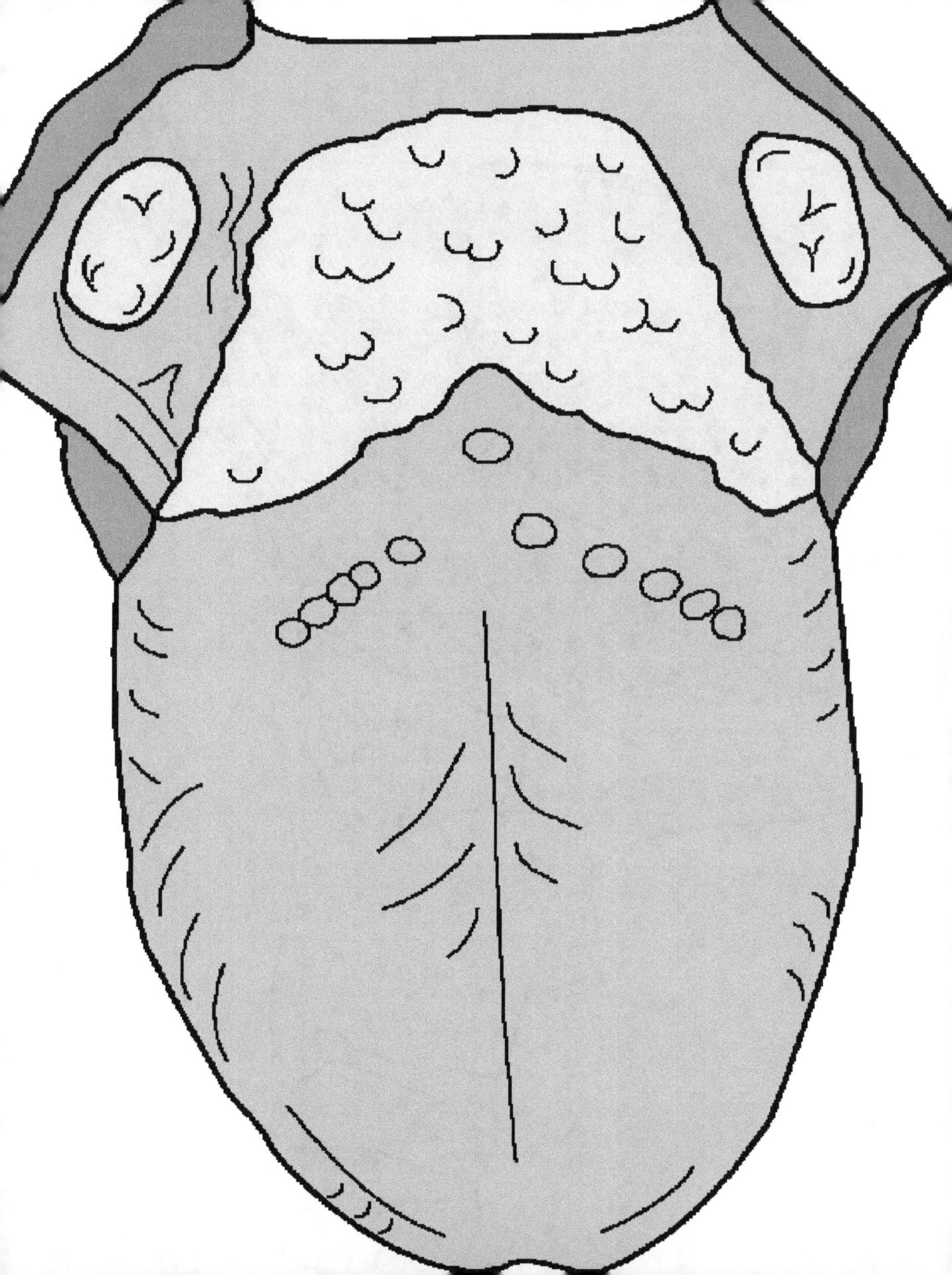

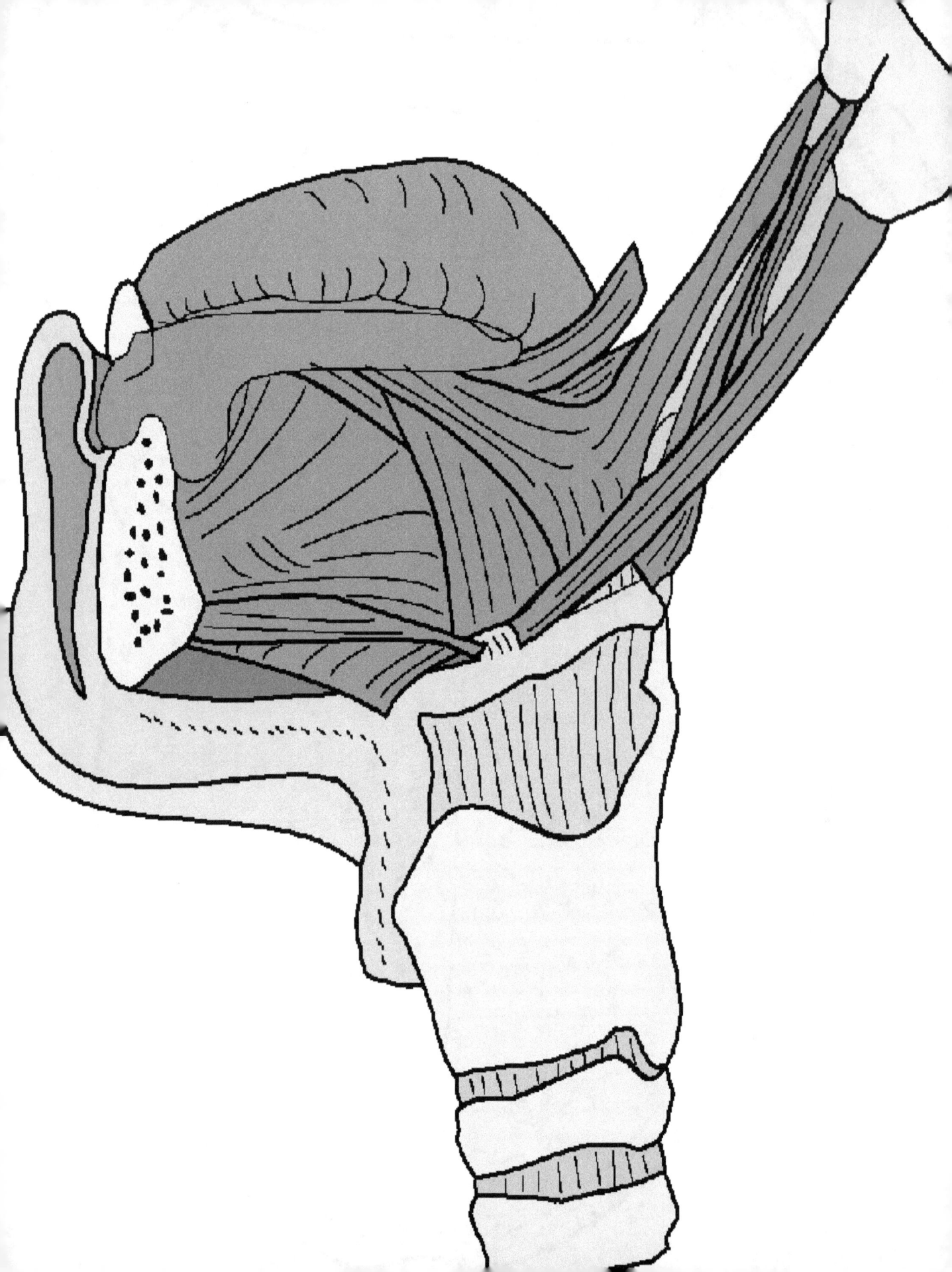

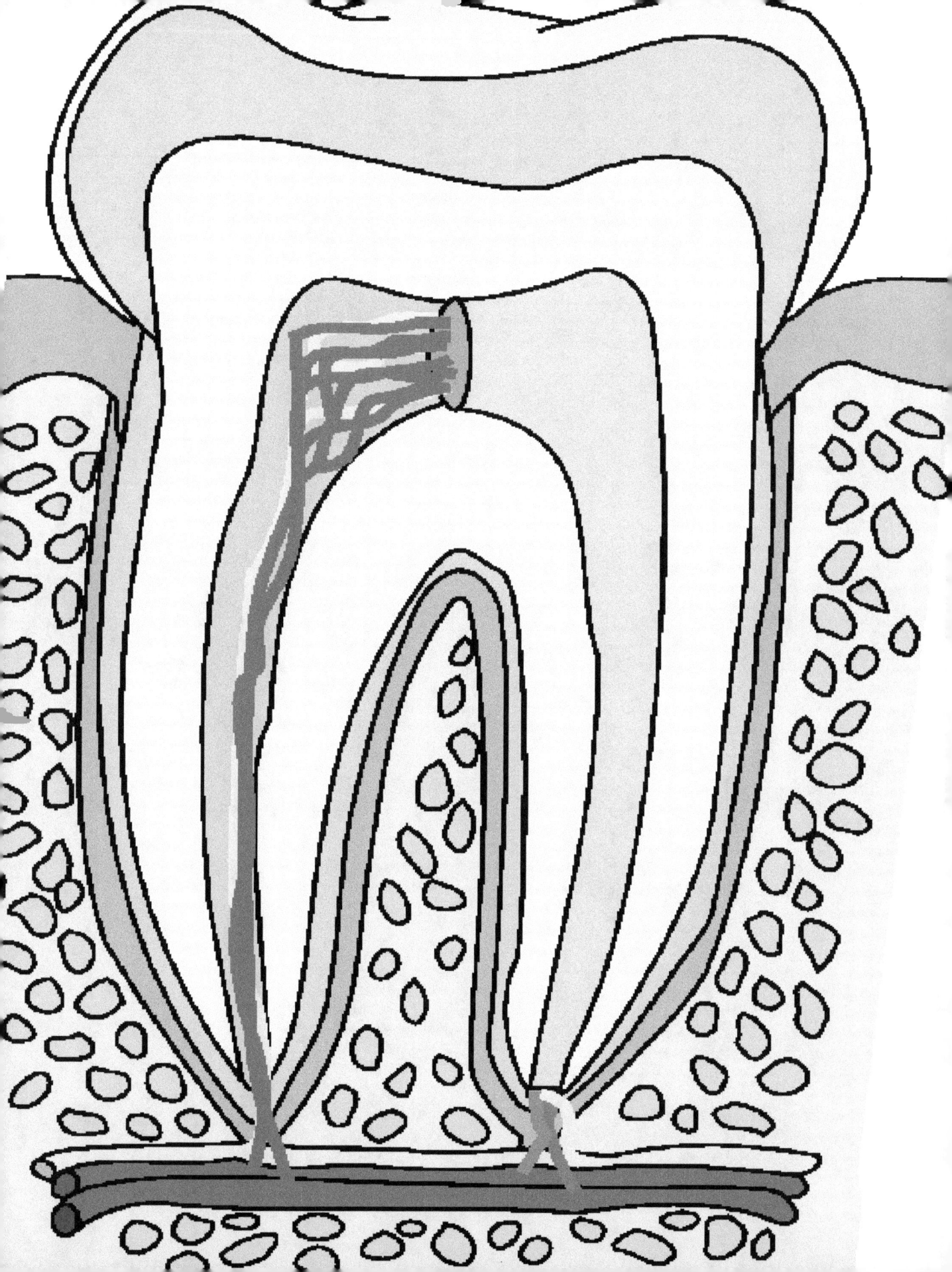

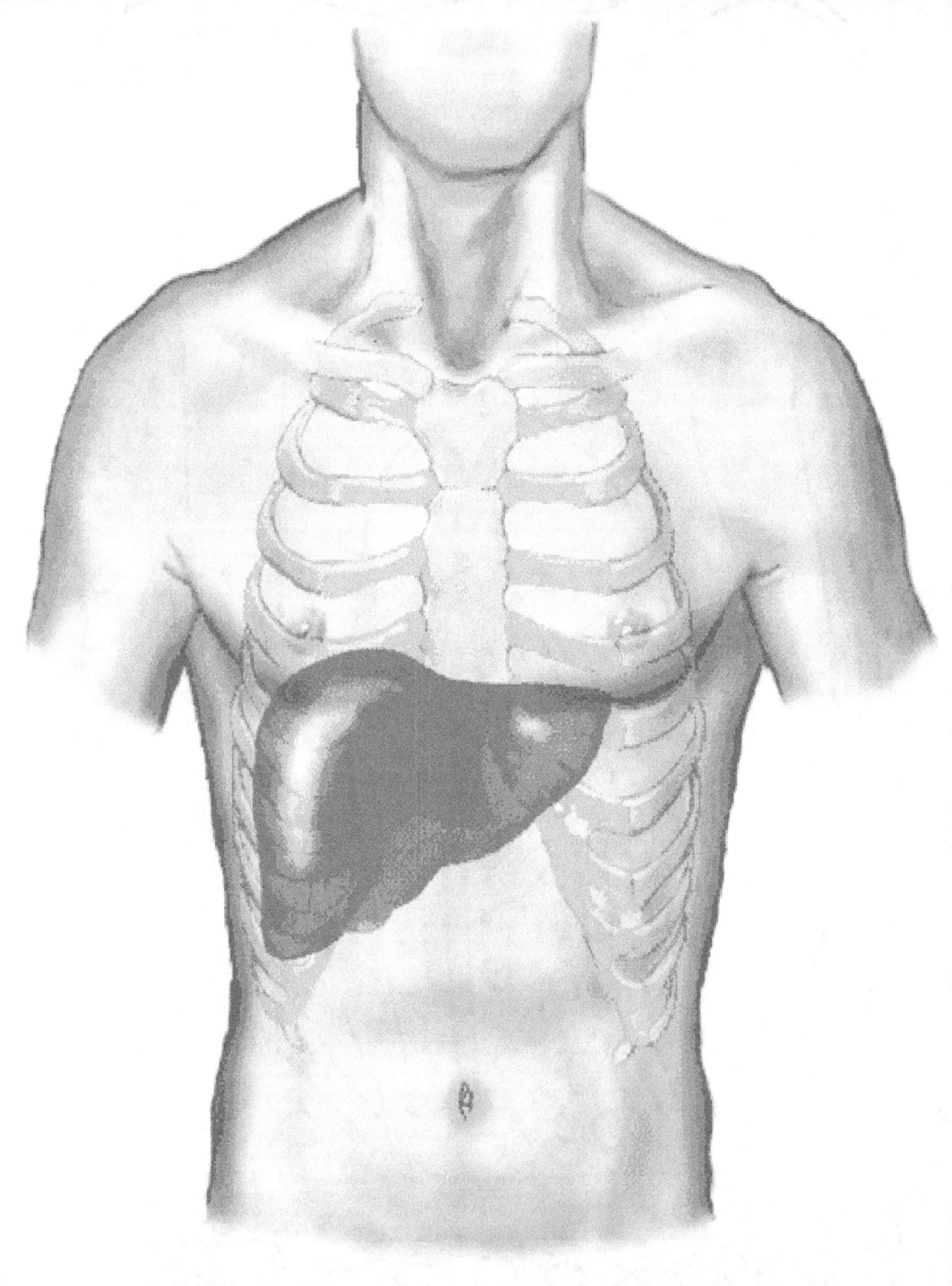

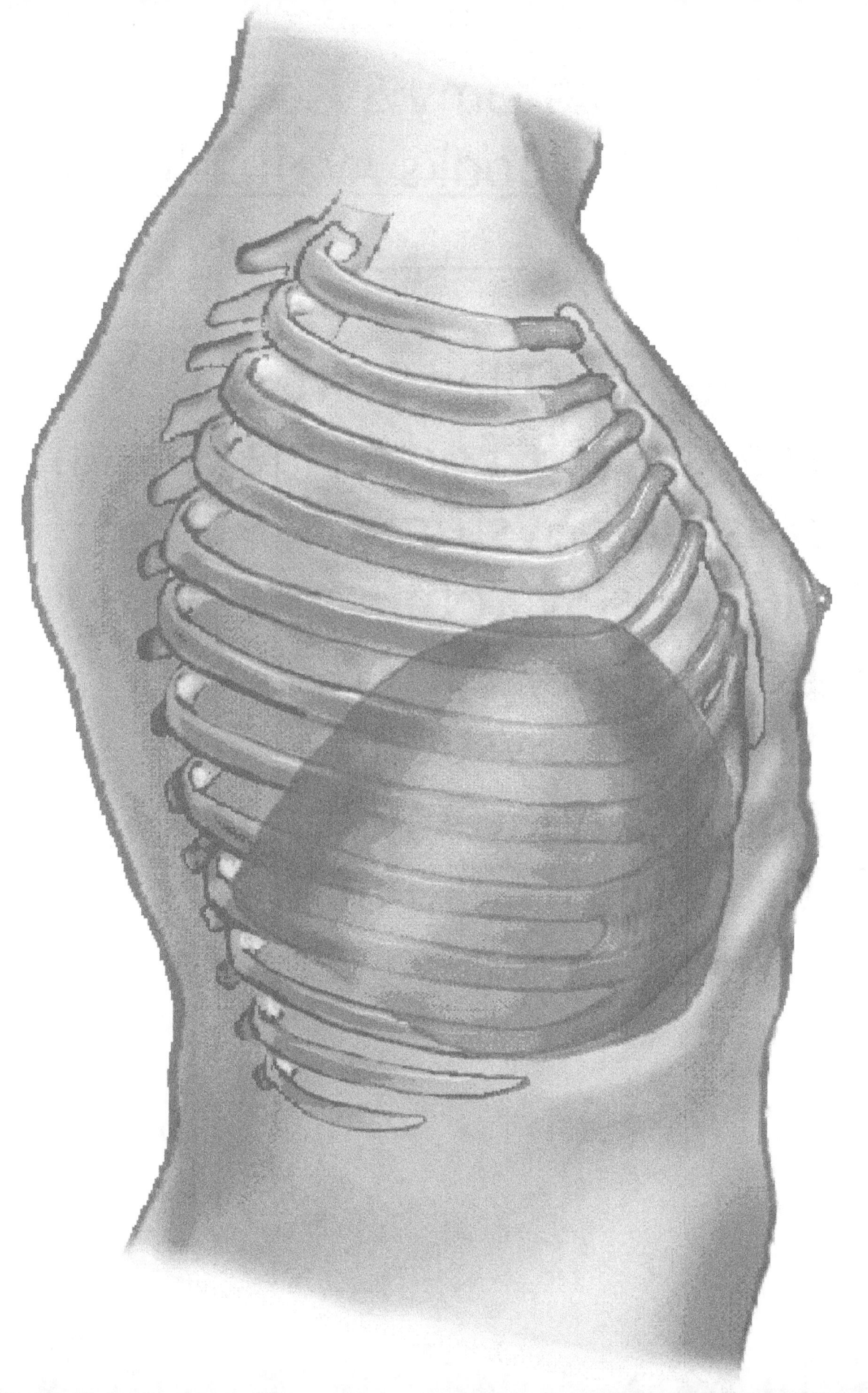

Other Anatomy System Label Practice <u>Books Available on</u>

<u>Amazon</u>

1. Cardiovascular System
2. Digestive & Endocrine System
3. Muscular System
4. Nervous System
5. Respiratory System
6. Skeleteal System
7. Surface Anatomy & Senses
8. Urogenital System

www.ingramcontent.com/pod-product-compliance
Lightning Source LLC
Chambersburg PA
CBHW080527190526
45169CB00008B/3081